I0759128

Fit & Fabulous

The No-Nonsense Approach to Controlling How You Age

PENELOPE LANE

Fit & Fabulous

The No-Nonsense Approach to Controlling How You Age.

Copyright @ 2023. Penelope Lane. All rights reserved. No part of this book may be reproduced by any mechanical, photographic, or electronic process, or in the form of a phonographic recording; nor may it be stored in a retrieval system, transmitted, or otherwise be copied for public or private use—other than for "fair use" as brief quotations embodied in articles and reviews—without prior written permission of the publisher.

This publication is designed to provide accurate and authoritative information regarding the subject matter covered. It is sold with the understanding that the publisher is not engaged in rendering legal, accounting, or other professional services. If you require legal advice or other expert assistance, you should seek the services of a competent professional.

Design and cover art by Jahz Rivera.

Disclaimer: The author makes no guarantees to the results you'll achieve by reading this book. All health improvement requires risk and hard work. The results and client case studies presented in this book represent results achieved working directly with the author. Your results may vary. See the Resources section for source citations.

Content

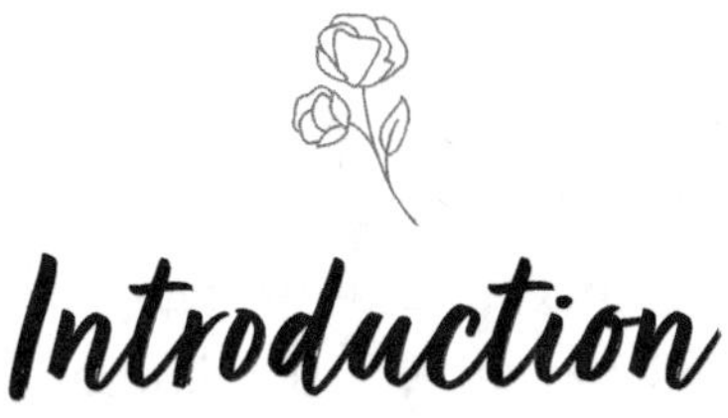

Introduction

No-nonsense aging is not a passive process.

This book is not about accepting your fate as you get older. It's about embracing the person you want to be and letting go of the stiff, frail, vague version of your-self life typically deals you.

It's also not about donning rose-coloured glasses and ignoring the fact that, yes, we are getting older.

One of my favorite go-to motivations comes from the Serenity Prayer:

Grant me the serenity to accept the things I can-not change, The courage to change the things I can, And wisdom to know the difference.

You are not too old to learn and understand and work within those things you have control over. Aging is not a hopeless process of loss and deterioration.

Believe it or not, there are so many more things you have control over than you don't, and that is an encouraging thought.

This book is written because I want to give you a space to know you are heard and validated. It really sucks to believe you've run out of time and you've lost all potential. I hope I can show you a different way.

My lived experience tells me there is a capacity within all of us to start living our lives a different way. It takes a lot of hard work, but magical things happen when we embrace four major principles of living and aging well.

These four principles are the pillars that inform not only the workouts I lead for women like you and me but also the attitude and practices I hope you adopt for a vibrant daily life.

There are a lot of books out there on weight loss, on exercise, and on the physical activities beneficial to your health. There are even books out there on aging gracefully, whatever that means for you.

There are very few, if any, books out there for us older folk that address the physical, cognitive, and emotional as they connect to a whole way of being.

My aim is to make this book as user-friendly as possible, providing connection, education, and simple practices that can drastically heighten the positives of your day-to-day life while allowing you to cope well with the negatives that will unquestioningly come.

I invite you to change how you relate to yourself, your health, and your overall well-being because there is real enjoyment to be had!

This is fun! It's bloody hard work, but it's fun bloody hard work.

I want you to age on your own terms so that you can keep doing those things that are important to you.

I want you to age on your own terms to benefit the people in your life that you love.

I want you to age on your own terms so you can create a ripple effect among your family, friends, colleagues, neighbors, and acquaintances.

If you take control of what you can - which I promise is more than you currently think you can! - its infectious nature will touch your spouse, your children, your grandchildren, your friends, and your neighbors.

I want you to age on your own terms to put a drop of goodness into the world and watch it continue on.

You can do this.

If all you get from this book is one thing, I want you to know that you can do something about your health and your future. You do not have to stay stuck. You do not have to simply wither and die.

My years of practicing clinical psychology and fitness training have combined to bring about this method of positive change. This beautiful realization that has rattled the cage of belief that I will slip into chronic illness and away from this earth; this understanding that, while I do not control the fact that I will age, I do have control over the way I age.

This method has provided me with confidence and the self-belief that I can age well and love the life I have left.

You don't have to live out your life feeling frail, sore, small, and ignored.

It doesn't have to be that way simply because that's what you've witnessed, told yourself, or heard from others.

I invite you to read with an open mind and heart to one simple truth: you can change the way you age.

If you'd like to meet with me, my door is always open. You are welcome to book an online chat with me at any time to explore your particular needs:

http://bit.ly/4br7lBz

Penelope

PART 1

Fit and Fabulous You

Chapter 1

What It Means to Be Fit and Fabulous

This book exists because I want you to feel you have a greater energy about you. It's physical, emotional, cognitive even. This energy is what allows you to do the things in your life that are important to you.

This is not about donning rose-coloured glasses. This is not a lecture about the things you have to do or that you should do.

This is about having the energy to embrace the demands in your life as well as the wishes in your heart.

This is about doing what you want more readily and easily without a second thought, whether that be going grocery shopping without a list because you remember what you need without it, being able to play with - or even pick up! - your grandchildren, or just keeping your sense of self intact with each passing year.

At this moment, in writing this book, I am 65 years old. The only illness I have is osteoporosis, bone deterioration, as a result of the neglect and abuse that happened when I dealt with anorexia and bulimia early in my life. Given the material in this book, I manage that significant health challenge through exercise.

At the age of 65, I don't get sick. I may have knocked on wood after writing that...but I just don't get sick. All through winter, my friends and family were dropping like flies. COVID made its rounds, and yet, I have maintained my health.

I have a sense that I am resilient. I am okay as a human being despite the fact that my inner critic is still there. She still talks to me, but she's muted. I don't worry too much about her to be honest.

I practice mindfulness and self-compassion in a way that I'm not trying to get rid of the negative parts of myself. I'd like to teach you to do the same. Instead of surgically removing them, the way I practice these principles merely changes my relationship with these critical parts of myself, so I have the capacity to mute them and go out into the world feeling that I am okay, that I am valuable, and that I have something to give.

My health and my mental well-being would all look vastly different without the principles and the methodology I live and thereby teach.

It may seem that considering principles like mindfulness, mood, self-confidence, and self-compassion can be ambiguous at best, but there are ways to measure your progress in these areas.

There is a daily check-in with a mindfulness practice that I do. The measurable factor there is my capacity to be mindful - present and aware - whilst I'm doing my practice and to be able to bring my attention gently back to what I'm focused on when I get distracted. I am content with my current pace, which is being mindful for most of 30 minutes each morning.

There are many studies that have been done on the benefits of the combination of mindfulness and self-compassion on overall well-being.

What's incredibly exciting is the newer research being done on the combined physical and cognitive training called dual tasking. This multi-component training is wonderful for many reasons, and it's a cornerstone of my programs and my life.

As you might expect, there are also measurable, quantifiable benefits to what I teach in relation to physical health. I've included one at the end of this chapter called The Step Test, and it's quite simple. You step up and down on a step for three minutes and then measure your heart rate. Over time, as you increase your fitness, your heart rate will get lower. If you'd like to compare notes, my heart rate with the step test is currently 86 bpm. I've been doing this for quite a long time, but that's a great indication of where you can get to, even at our age.

(In fact, once while having a procedure done at the hospital, the machine that keeps track of pulse kept beeping at the nurses that I might be dead because my resting pulse rate was so low! It's absolutely possible!)

There is also a newer branch in the world of physical exercise where movement (exercise) is being prescribed as a treatment for different chronic illnesses. In fact, your doctor, instead of prescribing (or in addition to) medication, could refer you to an exercise physiologist for prescriptive exercise to help with a chronic health condition. It's a wonderful addition to what we already understand about the human body and the benefits of exercise.

If you're interested, there are a couple of other physical tests you can perform to test your strength in your upper and lower body. I'll include those at the end of this chapter as well.

As an aside, you may scoff at my inclusion of strength training. That's for young guys trying to impress the good-looking girls at the gym, right? I want you to know that it is vital to your health, *especially as a woman*. Many women our age overlook strength training in favor of more cardio or maintaining flexibility. While heart health and limber muscles are great, please **do not discount what strength training can do for your health.** Even if you're dealing with arthritis or a chronic illness that makes it difficult, there are many low-impact options that can improve your strength and, thus, your overall health.

There's a phenomenon called sarcopenia, which is a horrible word, that means we lose muscle mass starting in our thirties. Strength training is critical to counteract this loss of muscle mass. Many people are aerobically inclined, but only 20% do strength training. Helping you get and stay strong and healthy is one of the main outcomes of my method.

This may all seem daunting. I often hear things like, "But I'm too old to start now," or, "I've lived this way for this long. It's fine." If you're having similar thoughts, take a look at the following case studies from women - just like you - who greatly improved their health and mental well-being in our work together.

Wendy Manages Pain and Gains Energy

Wendy found me through a Facebook Ad and was intrigued by an exercise class being run by an older woman. She felt I would understand her needs and, especially because I am a psychologist, that I would understand her.

Her goal was to change how she felt in her body and how she felt about her confidence, her relationship with herself. At the time, she was dealing with an inflammatory shoulder injury for which she was receiving regular cortisone shots when she first came to my classes.

She came to me, saying, "I don't have any fitness. I'm not fit. I don't have any energy. I'm tired all the time." It's a vicious cycle of not having cardio fitness. It makes you tired because everything else is just so much hard work. On top of that, enduring the bursitis in her shoulder, an injury brought on by strain, kept her in constant pain.

After several sessions, she wrote:

I haven't had any cortisone injections since we started working together. I just wanted you to know that. What you do is so important and just so valuable. It's the way you teach and the way you invite me to move my shoulders. You're always telling me what the alternative is during the workout. I can't lift my arms over my head, but you're always encouraging me. You're always getting me to keep moving by providing the alternatives, and you make me feel it's okay to do a different exercise to all the other women in the group. I don't feel uncomfortable that I have to do that. It's not that the pain has gone away. I just realised that I'm living with it so much better. I'm not investing in it being painful all of the time and then having to rush to the doctor every six months and have a cortisone injection.

I'm actually looking forward to hosting friends for Australia Day this year! For so many years, I would still do it, but I didn't look forward to it. I was so tired and had no energy, it was everything I could do just to show up. I now have more energy and I'm excited to host my friends. Thank you so very much.

Dorris Recovers From a Knee Replacement

Dorris found me when she was 8 months out of a knee replacement, and it was her second knee replacement. After her first knee replacement, her recovery went well. It took about six months and she could move around freely knowing everything was on the right path, but this knee replacement was different. She wasn't sure why, but it was taking so much longer to feel okay again.

When she first came to my classes, she would sit in a chair for any of the down-on-the-ground exercises. At the year mark of her second knee replacement, she was able to get down on the ground like everyone else in the class. The first time she was tentatively getting up, a few of us were poised around her, ready to help. She was fine with that, but when her husband went to help her, I encouraged him to let her do it on her own. Dorris said, "Yes, listen to Penelope. I want to do it on my own." And she did, to which we all gave a mighty congratulations!

Her goal was to be able to walk normally again. Knee replacements can change the way you walk, limit your movement, and increase your potential of falling over due to not only the physical aspects, but also the psychological lack of confidence in your movements and in your capacity to do daily activities. She came to me because, whilst other exercises were helping, she wanted my approach, knowing that it was about confidence, mindfulness, and the mind/body connection.

Lori Manages Early-Onset Alzheimer's Disease

Lori struggled with early-onset Alzheimer's Disease. She's been coming to my classes with her partner. She adores the classes and we adore her.

One of the signs of the cognitive deterioration common with Alzheimer's is losing the capacity to coordinate your body. One of the moves we do in our exercise group is getting on all fours and lifting the opposite arm and leg. (For example, lifting and extending your right arm and left leg at the same time.) In not being able to totally tell her body what to do, she would lift and extend the arm and leg on the same side – which is a feat in itself!

But now, I noticed that she is lifting and extending the opposite arm and leg. Lori is happy because she understands that this is a great achievement. Her capacity to command her body is improving, and she doesn't want me to make a big fuss of it, so I just give her a smile. She smiles back and knows that what she is doing is incredible.

She comes to the classes and tries everything. She hasn't given up or given in to her diagnosis. The classes have given her a way to slow the deterioration process and even improve her physical functioning.

What I'm sharing with you here is so much more than exercise. It's **connecting the body with the brain through movement whilst embracing the experience of what you're doing mindfully and learning to treat yourself like a good friend.**

This is a program that helps you develop an enjoyment of exercise. This is a program that takes the *whole* you into account, physically, cognitively, and emotionally, so you can get the best possible benefits for your health and well-being; *so you can keep doing what matters to you.*

Here's what I mean by "this is so much more than exercise."

What are the two core ingredients to develop an enjoyment of exercise?

1. The validation of the importance of it for your health.

2. The creation of the habit of just getting out there and doing exercise.

Seems pretty straightforward, but you've tried programs before that seemingly hit on both of these points, right? You know how important your health is. You may even avoid those thoughts and conversations because you're not sure how to reconcile your knowledge with your current habits. You've tried the calendars, the smart watches, the to-do lists, the walking groups, and the I'll-walk-the-dog-every-day attitude that lasts for a couple of months at best...

What you're missing are the elements of self-compassion, mindfulness, and cognitive training.

I'm absolutely serious. All of these aspects boost your

enjoyment, which brings satisfaction and, therefore, motivation. It's a beautiful cycle that doesn't start with berating yourself for not waking up to your alarm this morning to work out.

Most, if not all, women our age who are overweight or unfit are simply so because they haven't found something they can stick with. Nothing has worked or clicked for them. They've been waiting for some magical moment, a program or a pill or what have you, that will give them the motivation they need to stick to it.

It's not about a magic moment or program. It's about just coming at it from a different angle - and that different angle is developing mindfulness and self-compassion. Everything else naturally flows from there.

That's the lived experience that I have to share. When you develop mindfulness and self-compassion, combined with cognitive training and physical exercise, everything else falls into place. I am living proof of that.

Let's work through the assessments I've mentioned in this chapter:

- The Step Test: calculate your heart rate.

- Upper and Lower Body Strength: compare your results to the benchmarks included in the assessment.

- Self-Compassion Survey: this survey encompasses critical skills that are integral to your health.

Please take your time with each of these assessments as they will inform your true starting point and guide your progress in becoming your fit and fabulous self. Please pause the recording and get a piece of paper out so you can record your answers. And the assessments are on the website.

Self-Assessment #1: The Step Test

The step test is a great way to give you an estimate of your aerobic or cardio capacity. Follow the steps below to calculate your heart rate.

What you need for the test:

- You need a step around 30 cm high. You could use anything from a sturdy box to a concrete step.

- A timer of some kind.

The Step Test Process:

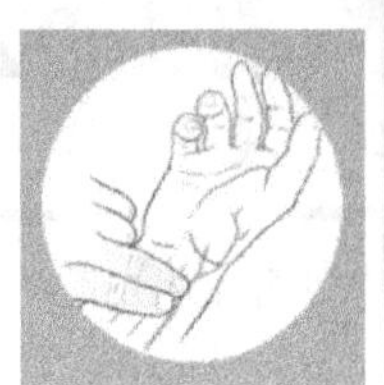

- Step up and down the step in the pattern left leg up, right leg up, left leg down, right leg down, etc.

- Do this at a steady pace, and maintain this pace through-out.

- After 3 minutes, stop

- Then, calculate your heart rate.

- You can measure your heart rate by counting the number of heartbeats inside one of your wrists.

- Count them for 15 seconds and then multiply by 4.

- The total amount is your heartbeat for 1 minute.

Self-Assessment #2: Upper and Lower Body Strength

Upper Body: Sit in a sturdy chair. You'll need one 2kg (4.4lbs.) dumbbell or other weighted object. Set a timer for 30 seconds. Count how many bicep (arm) curls you can do correctly before the timer expires. Be sure to fully extend your arm to a ninety-degree angle, all the way up, then back to ninety degrees.

Upper Body Strength Test Norms

Age	Average	Age	Average
55-60	14-20	75-79	11-17
60-64	13-19	80-84	10-16
65-69	12-18	85-89	10-15
70-74	12-17		

Lower Body: Set up a sturdy kitchen chair on a flat, non-slip surface with the back against a wall. Stand in front of the chair with your back facing it with your arms crossed at your chest. Set a timer for 30 seconds. Sit down and lightly touch the chair with your bottom and immediately stand up. Count the number of times you do this.

Lower Body Strength Test Norms

Age	Average	Age	Average
55-60	13-18	75-79	10-15
60-64	12-17	80-84	9-14
65-69	11-16	85-89	8-13
70-74	10-15		

Self-Assessment #3: Self-Compassion Survey

Below are statements about how you may typically act towards yourself in difficult times.

Using a scale from 1-5, please indicate how often you behave in the way described. Write your answer in the space provided next to each statement.

Please answer according to what really reflects your experience rather than what you think your experience should be.

1 = Almost Never

2 = Occasionally

3 = About Half of the Time

4 = Fairly Often

5 = Almost Always

	1. When I fail at something important to me, I become consumed by feelings of inadequacy.
	2. I try to be understanding and patient towards those aspects of my personality I don't like.
	3. When something painful happens, I try to take a balanced view of the situation.
	4. When I'm feeling down, I tend to feel like most other people are probably happier than I am.
	5. I try to see my failings as part of the human condition.
	6. When I'm going through a very hard time, I give myself the caring tenderness I need.

	7. When something upsets me, I try to keep my emotions in balance.
	8. When I fail at something that's important to me, I tend to feel alone in my failure.
	9. When I'm feeling down, I tend to obsess and fixate on everything that's wrong.
	10. When I feel inadequate in some way, I try to remind myself that feelings of inadequacy are shared by most people.
	11. I'm disapproving and judgemental about my own flaws and inadequacies.
	12. I'm intolerant and impatient towards those aspects of my personality I don't like.

Self-compassion is made up of self-kindness instead of self-judgment, common humanity instead of isolation, and mindfulness instead of over-identification.

Self-Compassion Scoring:

Self-Kindness

Add together questions 2 and 6. The higher the score, the more kind and friendly you are to yourself.

Self-Judgement

Add together questions 11 and 12. The higher the score, the more judgemental you are of yourself.

If you scored low in self-kindness and high in self-judgment, the best place to start is in being aware of your relationship to yourself. Keep reading and pay close attention to Chapters 6 and 7 and implement the self-compassion exercises in Part 3.

If you scored mid-line in both self-kindness and self-judgment, you're on your way there! Chapter 7 will give you a deeper look at self-compassion and Part 3 will give you exercises to try.

If you scored high in self-kindness and low in self-judgment, well done. You are doing a great job with this aspect of self-compassion. Check out Part 3 for additional exercises to try.

Common Humanity

Add together questions 5 and 10. The higher the score, the more you're able to sense that you share your concerns with others.

Isolation

Add together questions 4 and 8. The higher the score, the more lonely and isolated you feel when you're having problems.

If you scored low in common humanity and high in isolation, the best place to start is in learning how to be gentle with yourself while connecting with others. Read more about this in Chapters 6, 7, and 8. Then, pay particular attention to the exercises in Part 3.

If you scored mid-line in both common humanity and isolation, you are doing good, and there's room to improve. Look to the social aspects of self-compassion outlined in Chapters 7 and 8, then continue to Part 3 to continue on your way.

If you scored high in common humanity and low in isolation, you're doing a great job staying connected through your hard times. Way to go! If you'd like to work on this area any more, take a look at the exercises in Part 3.

Mindfulness

Add together questions 3 and 7. The higher the score, the more mindful you are in the way of accepting situations and being more balanced.

Over-identified

Add together questions 1 and 9. The higher the score, the more you tend to take things badly and personally when things aren't going well.

If you scored low in mindfulness and high in over-identification, the best place to start is learning about the connection your mind, body, and heart have as detailed in Chapter 4. After that, please continue through, paying particular attention to the mindfulness pillar in Chapter 7 and the mindfulness exercises in Part 3.

If you scored mid-line in mindfulness and over-identification, you've got a mindfulness skill that is still growing. Chapters 4 and 7 will deepen your understanding of mindfulness while the mindfulness exercises in Part 3 will guide you in your continued growth in this area.

If you scored high in mindfulness and low in over-identification, you've likely cultivated these skills mindfully - your hard work is showing. You may find Chapter 4 interesting, and Part 3 may have some exercises you can try if you'd like to add more to your practice of mindfulness.

. . . .

Thank you, Dr. Kristen Neff, whose amazing work I've drawn on to present this questionnaire.

Chapter 2

Taking Control of How You Age

What I'm really teaching you in the pages of this book is how to build your confidence and take control of the way your body and brain - both physiologically and psychologically - age.

The most powerful thing you can do to move forward is to be open to the prospect, to the idea, the belief that **you can take control of your health and well-being**.

You don't have to be at the mercy of the downward spiral of negativity and hopelessness that can be a part of the aging process. *You can, even at this point in your life and your health, affect significant changes to take charge of the way you age.*

My primary goal for you is to have an idea of what your day can look like, in terms of activity and personal reflection, so you can take control of the way you age and make those changes to your health and well-being. I want you to have a knowledge, an understanding, of what your life could look like and **then take the steps to put that knowledge into action**.

I've listened to and I've understood the many women, like you, that I've worked with. There are grandchildren to watch, children you're worried about, and not enough hours in the day. There's a sense that you've left the best of yourself behind and have fear of what's to come. I know many of you will want to discount what you read because you're dealing with chronic illness, pain, and other significant setbacks as a result of your age and your lifestyle.

I am 65 years old as I write this book. I am fit and healthy. I live a life full of vibrancy, but I wasn't always this way...

For the first 30 years of my life, I was overweight and totally shy. I lacked confidence, had mental health issues like anxiety and depression, and self-harmed. I felt like I wasted my late teens and all of my twenties as this time was dominated by self-hate, anorexia, anxiety, and bulimia. It's not like I'd experienced any trauma either. Far from it. I came from a loving family. It's just how things were for me at that time.

Perhaps because of my own suffering, I went to school and trained up as a psychologist. I graduated when I was pregnant with my son, who is now 35. When I got pregnant, I thought about exercising because my doctor said I was putting on too much weight with the pregnancy. For the health of my unborn child, I started swimming in the local pool, and for some reason it just clicked.

From that moment on, I was totally obsessed with exercise (in a good way!) and being the fittest and healthiest I could be for the pregnancy and subsequent birth of my son.

And I haven't stopped since then.

I even gave birth to my daughter 15 months later.

After that, I trained to become what was called a gym instructor (we didn't have personal trainers back then) and continued practicing as a psychologist. The three parallels, cognitive, physical, and emotional health, have been my obsession and love for 30+ years. At first, I just dabbled, teaching interested psychology clients in personal training sessions.

I am now retired from my private practice in clinical psychology, but I continue the combination of the cognitive, physical, and emotional because it works.

I spent the first half of my life unfit, lacking confidence, feeling a great lot of shame, certainly not having any resilience, not feeling strong or capable, and being very self-critical. I wonder if you can relate to any of these.

For whatever reason, pregnancy was a magic bullet. It was like there was something more than just me and I wanted to be as fit and healthy as possible. The rest is history. I have lived my life with a strong foundation of knowing the benefits from combining physical, cognitive, and emotional health. This is where the four-pillar approach was born.

I am here to help you experience those same benefits. Being healthy for my family has made all the difference in the world.

There are a lot of lovely, nubile, young people promising results online. That's great, but I'm here specifically for the 50, 60, 70, and 80-year-old women who are - or want to be - active.

I am not a chair exercise person. This is not a chair-based program. If you want to work with me, you'll need to be mobile and reasonably active (even if that just means you enjoy a good walk around the block).

This is for you if you've tried the gym and, for whatever reason, it's just not for you. You've perhaps tried some online programs, but it's difficult to stick with.

If you're looking for something that will help you start something, enjoy the process, and get - and maintain - benefits quickly, I can help you.

As I presented this to one client, her response was, "Oh, I guess I am 60, huh?"

I want to reach out to the women reading this who may intellectually know their age but aren't embracing it and who aren't taking up the challenge of doing what they can to take control of how they age. We grow up in a society where we fear getting old and for good reason. As we say to our grandkids, getting older isn't for sissies!

But I encourage you to consider... What do you want your life to look like at 60? At 70? 80? 90? Getting older can mean different things to you based on your life experience and personality.

You can decide how you want to dress, act, and show up to your life. Define that for yourself. Do you want to be the grandma who attends your grandchild's sports events wearing their team colors, even if it's not really your color, and shouting the loudest from the sidelines? Embrace it! Do you want to be the neighbor known for the world's most moist carrot cake? Go for it!

Define, determine, and then act upon what your 60-years-old and beyond is going to look like.

I have been gray since I was 30-years-old, and I dyed my hair right up until I was 56. One day, I just refused to dye my hair anymore. Aside from all of the chemicals in hair dye, I felt it was unnecessary, but it was a pivotal moment for me because I know what being gray meant in our society. It's changing slightly because of people who are embracing their gray, but it was a real act of self-validation, self-kindness, and self-care.

We'll talk more about this later, but it's more about how you relate to yourself than anything else.

I wanted my 60s and beyond to mean I was strong, and I am. I am physically strong because of exercise. I am mentally and cognitively strong because of mindfulness and cognitive training. I am emotionally strong because of the self-compassion I practice. It's not magic. It's not that I was blessed by anything. It's because of the techniques I use, the very same techniques I'm here to teach you.

I've been combining psychology and fitness for a long time. I'm practiced, researched, and passionate about helping the women I teach.

Chapter 3

Outside of Your Comfort Zone

I feel like I can tell you that I know what you're thinking. It's difficult to hear promises like the ones I'm making and not automatically ask for the catch.

In this chapter, I want to address the top things that can get in the way of my clients considering doing something outside of their current comfort zone. I call these hindrances.

For each outlined hindrance, I will also briefly explain how my approach helps to address that specific hardship or situation.

Let's get started!

Hindrance #1: Lack of Self-Belief

If you don't *believe* that you can have the health and well-being that you want to, that belief will act as a solid brick wall, a thick, steel edifice, and stop you in your tracks.

It's impenetrable. No matter how many times someone says to you, "Oh, don't be silly. You can [do that thing] or [learn that skill]." Or, better yet, "It's okay. I can help you." – they cannot break through that wall of a lack of self-belief.

It completely gets in the way. No matter how much compassion comes to you from others who have your best interests at heart, it's hard to get around that lack of self-belief. Even if you tend to come from the other direction, you know that a tough-love approach - criticism or a kick in the behind - will not push you past that lack of self-belief.

Are you listening more to your inner critic than your inner supporter?

Women who lack this vital aspect of self-belief tend to speak more negatively about themselves and others. We all have an inner critic, but lacking self-belief gives that inner critic more power. When they describe something, particularly about themselves, that they've been able to do in their lives or that they want to do in their lives, it is couched in negativity and doubt. There's a sense of wanting those things, but they don't think they'll ever be able to do those things, and no one can tell them otherwise. While they would say they want to be optimistic, there's a sure tendency towards pessimism. Many of the women I encounter have the glass-half-empty outlook mixed with this incredible angst and shame that "things can't be, in any way, different" for them.

Do you identify with this hindrance to your health and well-being?

If so, you're not alone! This is number one on the list because of its prevalence. It makes perfect sense that you feel this way.

We watched our mothers, the 50s and 60s generation, who didn't have a choice but to be subservient to everyone else around them. It was just how things were.

My own mother - who is currently 91 - was very avant-garde when we were small. She worked in a professional career position but would still come home after working eight hours and clean the house and cook dinner every night (and I might add that dinner was always a three-course meal).

This is what many women grew up watching as normal. Dad ruled the house, plain and simple.

Then, we had women like Oprah, Louise Hayes, or Brené Brown (though she's more modern) - and some blokes in the mix as well. They invited women to question how they were living their lives. They asked us to explore how we related to ourselves, particularly how we talked to ourselves about ourselves and the beliefs we had around who we were as people and as women.

This awareness turns out to be key to our good health and well-being...but how you put that awareness into positive action was still a mystery. It still is for many of us.

We're told to start looking after ourselves, to go and have a massage, grab coffee with a friend, or take a nice hot bath. None of that is wrong, by the way. Those are wonderfully nurturing activities. The issue is that looking after themselves stops there - after the bath or massage or what-have-you. It's really lovely while you're in the bath or getting the massage, but when you step back into your life, you're back to all of the same habits of how we talk to ourselves and the same lack of self-belief.

Our proclaimed self-care doesn't reach as far down as it needs to in order to affect real change in our overall health.

There is comfort around doing those self-care tasks like having a massage and a bath, but the key is to feel okay about it afterward. Our generation has an awareness that we're beating ourselves up or giving ourselves a hard time, but we haven't really been taught what to do about that. We certainly haven't been taught how to make a permanent, life-changing difference in how we relate to ourselves.

The nuts and bolts you need to relate to yourself in a compassionate way, as you would with a friend, is what I teach within the self-compassion pillar of my framework. The seed of self-compassion is in the exercise workouts I teach. You want self-compassion to become integrated into your life as you live it.

In my program, you apply this principle of self-compassion to specific tasks you do every day.

The growth of self-compassion flows into developing a friendlier relationship with your own self, which enhances your self-belief and worth.

*H*indrance #2: Lack of Trust

You know me at least well enough to buy my book... but chances are, there is still a lack of trust.

Younger people don't feel as much of a barrier between an online persona and themselves as we oldies do. The connections with people we only know virtually are not part of our conditioning, not part of our lived experience. It's difficult to trust someone you can't actually physically connect with.

You're wary of being sold to, which, let's be honest, is all over the place.

The only reason you're willing to put up with it here is because I'm sharing something with you, something you desire: help and encouragement towards a result you want in your life.

Want to know my secret angle? Are you looking for the fine print? Here it is: I'm telling you everything I know in this short book because I value the importance of helping others when I can. I trust that there are women who will want more help implementing what they learn, and I want to make it as easy as possible for those women to raise their hands and get my help.

If you're not one of those women, that's okay! Keep reading. The information you need is all here. You've made a commitment to buy my book, so it's very important to me that you get something good in return.

I know you're much more comfortable in a small setting: coffee with a friend, chatting in a group, going to a hobby-based activity group, etc.

The truth is, being online isn't easy for me either, *but it's where I need to be in order to reach the women I want to teach.*

So, if you want to meet me, book a coffee chat time here for a quick meetup on Zoom:

http://bit.ly/4br7lBz. I value this face-to-face time so much. I make this a regular part of my program. My group meets, in person and virtually, for coffee after some of my workouts because _connection is a primary driving force behind the results we get with my method._

It's the connections in our lives that are motivating to us in the first place: wanting quality time with our partners, wanting to be around for our children, wanting to get on the floor and play with our grand-children, wanting to be healthy enough to take care of elderly parents, wanting to be strong and switched on enough for our own sake...

Connection drives us.This book is my rebellion against the social media age we live in, against the hard sells and empty promises so prevalent in our world. Spend some time with me in the pages of my book whilst learning the basics so you can bolster your health and well-being.

I'm here to meet you where you are, wherever you are, to help you on your way to healthy habits and self-sufficient, active aging.

I'm serious about the offer for a Zoom coffee chat: _http://bit.ly/4br7lBz_

Hindrance #3: I'm Too Busy

A busy and frantic life isn't unfamiliar to you. There are many demands on your time.

At our age, we're caught between caring for our elderly parents, supporting our children, and trying to spend as much time with our grandchildren as we can.

Even if those scenarios don't apply to you, there are doctor's appointments, social relationships, and even jobs.

We are very much sandwiched between the older and younger generations. It's really difficult because we grew up to believe that when we retired, we were going to go off and travel and do all of these lovely, creative, and feel-good things for ourselves, but that's not turning out as we thought it would for many different reasons.

We are a generation that knows it's important to factor in self-care, but we don't because we're too busy, and everyone else still comes first.

I am familiar with the frenetic energy that can accompany this time in life. There are last minute things that pop up and, suddenly, you can't do that thing you wanted to do for yourself today. There's disappointment, anger, annoyance, resentment, and/or guilt.

Nothing is really as you pictured it would be.

Life happens. Mothers fall over, fathers get ill, children desperately need your help, and today, there's no way around it. Of course it is necessary to drop everything to take care of other people in our lives.

The difference I want you to experience is after the storm has passed. You're not going to then beat yourself up because of the other things that fell off of your plate. You'll learn how to factor in the stuff that's outside of your control and adjust, looking forward to tomorrow.

If you carry on with the full program, you'll create the intention to affirm you can and will create the time to do three 30-40 minute workouts each week. If you make the choice to be involved in the program, you'll receive the exact tools you need to change the relationship with yourself and your own self-belief *so you can prioritize your needs amongst all of the other things you need to do.* Being active three times a week with my unique workouts is part of that.

The discipline required soaks into other areas of how you live your life, creating the foundations for no-nonsense aging.

*H*indrance #4: Household Budget

I want to first off recognize that not everyone is in a position to fund self-investment, and I'm not here to tell you otherwise. You know your financial situation better than anyone, most of all me.

What I can tell you is that I know how it feels to consider investing in myself. It can feel foreign. It can give you sleepless nights and leave you agonizing over whether the money is really worth it. Couldn't you just carry on as you have been?

There's a bit of an angst and anxiety around these thoughts because, deep down, we know the value. If we didn't, we wouldn't give it a second thought. Think of all the things presented to you every day. You don't notice all of those things. If you notice something, it means that it resonated with you on a subconscious level and that, deep down, that thing is important to you. More often than not, our self-doubt and fear get in the way of us experiencing what really matters to us.

So, all I can offer you is what I do when faced with a tough financial decision.

When my head is telling me something is too expensive, I feel into and mull over the actual value of a thing for me personally.

What am I actually getting here?

What changes will it actually bring about? Why is that important?

Will it add value to other people in my life as well as myself?

Answer these questions objectively and specifically. This is the matrix I used when investing in a program to grow my business and when getting this book written and into your hands. I understood specifically what I was receiving, the changes it would affect in my business and my life, why it's important to me to grow and help more women, and the value it will add to others in my life, including you.

My mum used to tell me that if you buy cheap things, you're going to get cheap things - and they'll break or stop working. I remember my parents always bought quality furniture. They didn't own any cheap furniture. Both of my parents worked and they bought lovely, home-crafted Jarrah things. (That's the wood here in Australia.) They invested well to reap the benefits for years to come.

One last question to consider: is there a cost to not participate? Does the cost of not participating shift the scales for you? Everyone's answer will be different, and only you can determine what feels right for you. I know for myself, the cost of not investing in a program to grow my business meant a future life living on a pension with no assets to provide the buffer required for a comfortable and happy existence.

If you need more information about my program to help you answer the above questions, you can reach out to me _here_. I hope you understand by now that I'm not into hard-selling. I want you to make the best choice for you, and only you know what that is.

Hindrance #5: How Is This Going to Be Different for Me?

I know you have a lot of lived experiences and have heard of or participated in many programs and promises that fell flat in comparison to your expectations.

How do you know I'm not packaging up the same things you've tried before?

1. I haven't always been how I am now. You may recall my story from Chapter 2. My lived experience is what I am teaching: that this works. In fact, I won't talk about or sell anything I haven't experienced for myself.

    When I was a psychologist, there was always a new technique that would come out (as there always is), but I would always go back to the mindfulness-based cognitive therapies because I knew that worked for me personally.

I knew it worked for my clients. I knew the research behind it. I will only teach what resonates with me.

2. I stay on top of the research, utilizing meta-analyses[1] (where the results from various studies in one area are compiled into a conclusion). I do this in the fields of exercise, mindfulness, self-compassion, and cognitive training (the four pillars of my program, which we'll get much more into later in this book).

3. I have years of experience with women in my exercise groups, my psychology groups, my mindfulness groups, and now my combined exercise and cognitive training groups. I know, not just by my feeling from working with women for so long but in all of the lovely feedback they give me. It's normally like pulling teeth to get reviews, but the spontaneous feedback is richer and deeper anyway.

When we meet for our virtual or in-person coffee after our classes, I take in little things they say, I hear the lovely conversations, and it's so invaluable. I know this is changing their lives and helping them to stay in control of how they're aging and showing up in their lives.

---

[1] *See the References Section for a list of meta-analyses supporting the content in this book.*

Anything you read in this book has gone through each of these three gates: my lived experience, research, and client success. Anything I sell is based on these three principles: I've tried it for myself, I've done extensive research in my professional fields and stay up-to-date on new techniques and what works, and I have years of working with women just like you.

Fear of the unknown can stop you in your tracks. It can stop you from trying something new. It's uncomfortable to try, especially when you have good excuses! You're too busy, you're sore, you've got that injury, you're tired, you're overwhelmed, and you're just struggling in your life. Feeling fear is a comfort, in a way, as it keeps you safe in what you know and what's familiar, even if it's not serving you well or helping you.

I encourage you to start with what you see, hear, and feel from all that I've shared with you here in this book. Give yourself the benefit of experiencing the principles you learn here firsthand. Take it one step at a time. Be kind to yourself. Be open to how much of a difference this can make.

One solid, fundamental principle my teaching is based on involves the interconnectedness of the brain, body, and heart and that you treat yourself as whole.

Chapter 4

Mind, Body,
and Heart

We aren't only our minds, we aren't only our bodies, and we aren't only our feelings. We are all of these combined.

There isn't actually a mind separate from your body and separate from your heart. It's just one thing, reallyly. That's the essence of my approach.

We are not these things as separate entities (as most of us have been taught).

Understanding this critical truth is the "secret" to success in aging on your own terms. Separating the body, mind, and heart only creates the illusion of more; more problems to deal with in the present moment, more to keep up with for a healthy life, and more items on a to-do list already longer than Santa's present list.

Mind, body, and heart are interconnected. Improving one area impacts the other two every time. When examined closely, each pair reveals undeniable laws that can help us in our quest to age on our own terms.

Mind and Body

The first - and often easiest - to see is the connection between our minds and our bodies.

The technical scientific term is **proprioception**.

This connection gives us the sense of being able to move our bodies without having to consciously think about it, like picking up a glass of water, walking up or down the stairs, or talking with your hands.

When you're on a walk with a friend, you don't focus on each and every step. You're able to walk along and direct your attention to the conversation instead of concentrating on each step you take.

Can you imagine a day (or even five minutes!) without this proprioception?

You would be thinking about every movement in detail. "I'm going to move my arm up, wave my fingers, and put my arm down. Alright, now I'm going to move my hand up - good! - now back down."

How exhausting that would be! We would need more naps without our proprioception guiding those automatic movements.

This mind-body connection can deteriorate.It can become fractured by age, tiredness, depression, chronic illness, or inflammation. The connections in our brains that drive this action without conscious effort fray, leaving the mind wanting more direction. For example, fractured proprioception is one of the reasons people trip and fall over. As we get older, there is so much more concentration that has to go into putting one foot in front of the other. Walking up stairs is a deliberate act instead of the mindless activity most of us experience.

When an individual experiences fractured or compromised proprioception, they need more forethought to engage in regular, everyday activities like walking, speaking, eating, etc.

It is important to keep working this connection between mind (brain) and body like we would any muscle. We need to keep training it to respond. The myth that our proprioception will keep on working regardless of what we do is false. We need to consciously and actively engage our mind-body connection.

Continually working this mind-body connection gives us the best possible shot of living our lives naturally and normally for as long and as best as we can.

One of the exercises we use in my program that is very helpful focuses on slowing our walking gait.

Each step gets broken into three parts: heel, ball, toe.

You place your heel on the ground first, then shift forward to the ball of your foot, and end with your toes on the ground. By breaking this into three parts, you are more aware and deliberate about your movement forward. The mind-body instruction here is being intentional and mindful of the feeling of each part of your step.

Then, we go in reverse: toe, ball, heel.

This is where participants start to feel the efficacy of this exercise. In fact, this is a common exercise among our generation simply because there is little to equal how well this works in maintaining - and even improving - the connection between mind and body.

So, if you've recently had a fall or you notice that you've had to concentrate more while walking on the stairs or which way the door goes when you open it - things we take for granted - this type of mind-body training is incredibly helpful. It rewires parts of the brain that were present before and have just gotten fractured and disconnected over time.

The good news is that you don't have to put up with this forever! You can actually retrain your proprioception - as long as you haven't had a traumatic brain injury or anything like that. All being well in the brain, you can actually rewire those same connections that were there before.

Mind and Heart

In this sense, we're not referring to your heart as in your cardiac health - your heart means your emotion. In essence, there is a connection between your thoughts and your feelings.

The thousands of everyday thoughts we experience influence how we feel. If we have a negative thought, we are going to tend toward feeling negative emotion.

We're often given the advice to think happier thoughts or practice gratitude to lift our spirits on a down day. Now, it's not as simple as "think positive, feel positive," but it's a start to understanding that our thoughts or cognitions affect our emotional experiences.

How your mind works very much influences your emotional experience of the present moment.

Some people explain it by saying, "I just suddenly felt

sad," or, "I quickly reacted in anger. I didn't even think about it." While that might explain the experience you had, there is still a thought that comes before the emotion.

Many of us relate to the world through an emotional lens. That's what we pay attention to or what's most important to us. Before an emotion erupts in our hearts, there is a cognitive process that takes place. Something happens, and there is a quick interpretation in terms of what that event meant to you - and it's more likely to be unconscious. Then follows the emotional reaction, whether that emotion is felt only internally or explodes into our words and actions.

In my experience of working with women over these many years, emotion doesn't happen automatically. There is a thought, a process, and a trigger that instigates the emotion.

The process starts in the mind and travels to the heart. There is something internal or external that has happened, then we have a thought about it. We interpret, assume, or expect - all activities of the mind - in order to have an emotional experience tied to that initial event.

I am sometimes flabbergasted at how we are generally taught about this connection. Well-meaning advice can sound like:

"Don't be sad, darling."

"Put on a smile. Be happy."

"It'll be okay. Just forget about it."

"Here, have an ice cream. That will make you feel better."

These were commonly given to us as children and are often something we're guilty of saying to our children, our grandkids, or ourselves.

The focus is put on changing or trying to stop the emotion without addressing the impetus of these feelings: our thought processes.

Teaching this awareness of thoughts is a key part of what I teach, reinforcing an awareness of the connection between mind and heart instead of treating them as separate entities.

This training is essential to navigating the aging process in a graceful and empowered way so you can cultivate a vibrant life.

Body and Heart

Whatever happens in the body influences your emotions.

The best example of this is pain.

Pain is a physical experience. We twist our ankles or

deal with chronic pain like arthritis, and there's an experience of pain. We don't like pain. It hurts.

Our minds chime in and say, "Oh, that's awful. I don't like that." Then, we feel emotions like frustration and avoidance, not wanting to feel the pain. Then, we have the pain to deal with and the added burden and discomfort of avoidance. That makes us feel even worse and can also make the pain much worse.

We then feel down, sad, or even angry when we're in pain, even if you wouldn't categorize an experience as painful - feeling achy or sore comes with the same natural inclination of avoidance and resistance. If it's unpleasant, we resist it, making us feel worse.

In this way, pain is a wonderful example to teach us that what happens in the body influences us emotionally. Physical experiences trigger emotional experiences. Fuelled by thoughts, perceptions of physical experiences to the emotional ones.

Of course, the opposite side of the coin is just as applicable here. If we experience something in the body like a nice meal, a massage, or a soothing touch on the shoulder, we feel uplifted and positive emotions surrounding those events.

Your mind, body, and heart are intricately and inseparably connected.

Mind, Body, and Heart Combined

You are mind, body, and heart, inseparably connected.

You are whole. This is the idea behind my entire methodology. Without understanding this essential, foundational principle, aging on your own terms be-comes a laborious task - and often feels out of reach. Approach yourself with the understanding that your mind, body, and heart are interconnected and you are well on your way.

One of the first steps to embracing this concept is this idea that you can step back and distance your-self from an experience you don't like. That could be negative thoughts, troubling emotions like guilt or a sense of shame, or pain and discomfort in the body.

This is the skill of awareness where you become an observer to your own experiences. You cultivate a ca-pacity to separate yourself from negative experiences and become aware of what is actually happening in the present moment. This doesn't mean you're sitting there zen-like and zoned out. It means you're actually more connected to what you are experiencing in your mind, body, and heart.

This skill falls under a larger umbrella of a main pillar I'll go further into later (in Chapter 7) called *mindful-ness*.

You'll learn how to be aware of your thoughts, observe what emotions those thoughts rouse, and identify what physical sensations accompany your thoughts and feelings.

When you are lost in the murky weeds - a strong emotion, incessant thought, or painful physical experience - there is little awareness of the big picture. You're unable to identify any surrounding details that could be helpful because you're too close, too involved in the initial experience. This is what is meant by "you become your thoughts" or "you become your emotions."

You can feel tossed to and fro between your thoughts, feelings, and experiences. Mindfulness keeps you grounded.

Becoming an observer doesn't mean you're unable to feel and respond. It doesn't mean you don't have bad days or strong feelings. It means that when you feel angry, you understand that you are a person experiencing anger as opposed to labeling yourself as an angry person or that you experience anxiety or sadness versus labeling yourself as an anxious or sad person.

When you feel unmotivated and disappointed, you are able to weather the put-downs you place on yourself because, as an observer, you're able to take a step back and understand the other aspects that play into your current lack of drive.

Practicing this crucial skill of taking a step back and observing rather than reacting is the gateway to real and lasting self-improvement because you're not lost in the mire and hopelessness of being an angry person, a sad person, an anxious person, or a lazy person. You experience an openness and freedom to see how you can make things different in your life. This is half of the change that allows you to live how you want to as you age, and it encompasses two of the four pillars imperative to your aging health: mindfulness, which we've touched on, which leads to self-compassion. Both of these will be explored in more detail in Chapter 7.

Cultivation of the mind, body, and heart connection allows you to become more aware and focused on yourself in a productive way. Observing all of those experiences from an outside perspective means you can do something about it. You are not the stuff of life because you are not bogged down with all the emotion. You are separate from it. You can see the entire forest instead of a few of the trees.

This takes several skills I will cover later, but know that this can't be an intellectual exercise. You can't just read a book or an article or have someone sit you down and tell you how it works. You have to actually try your hand at it and experience and develop your own internal 'observer.'

This is a large part of what I teach. The women I work with develop a strong sense of who they are. From that grounded place - and with lots of practice! - they are able to distinguish between the thoughts, emotions, or physical sensations they experience and know they are separate from these experiences. This heightened awareness gets to such a level, degree, and depth so they can then do something about what they are experiencing. *It is this seemingly simple but crucial skill that allows them to be as healthy as possible as they get older - that allows every woman to age on their own terms.*

If this sounds impossible right now, that's okay. I detail the specific pillars of my methodology and give you specific first steps to take, so even if we don't get the chance to work together, you can benefit. You are not doomed to a downward spiral of aging. You can infuse this chapter of your life with health, well-being, strength, and vibrancy - it's not too late!

Chapter 5

Common Health Worries of Aging

As you get older, the chances of having age-related pain increases. The main reason is one you've been aware of since your mid-thirties: the body doesn't work as well as it did when it was younger.

There's a sort of "use by" date in the sense of having our bodies working optimally. We're not trying to reverse this. You can't reverse it. It's important to embrace this concept as we get older to work within and beyond the changes we experience in our bodies.

Rather than getting lost and locked in to "I can't do anything about this," we learn to say, "Here is what is happening to my body. What can I do about it?" We search for the things that help and embrace what you find that resonates with you, especially because you need to understand that *your aging body is not your fault*.

You are getting older. Every year, your body ages a little more. That is the natural way of things. That is true. It is also true that having joint pain or chronic illness is not a punishment for sitting too long or not looking after yourself. It's not a given that you must endure joint pain or chronic illness simply because you are old. We'll talk a little more about this in the next chapter.

For now, I want you to know that it's not your fault that your body is aging and that there is absolutely a way to be proactive about your health within the experiences and limitations of your age.

Simple, age-related wear and tear on the body can create soreness, discomfort, stiffness, and it can even create pain. Within our collective aging experiences, the two most common ailments are chronic illnesses and arthritis.

Arthritis

I mainly work with women who experience osteoarthritis, primarily caused through wear and tear in the aging process. There is another type of arthritis called rheumatoid arthritis, which is an autoimmune response. There are differences in how these types of arthritis are experienced and addressed, though the basics we discuss here will be helpful to those experiencing either type of arthritis.

The main cause of arthritis is inflammation brought on by a number of different factors, wear and tear to joints being the main one. Lifestyle factors also play a role, like a poor diet and chronic stress. The go-to treatment for arthritis is anti-inflammatory medications. Those can be helpful, sure, but the heart of the matter lies in movement, activity, or exercise.

I know this sounds counterintuitive. Why would you want to move when it's painful to do so?

I will teach more about arthritis in Chapter 7. What I want to impress upon you at this point is that I get it. Being in pain is hard, and moving through that pain is even harder.

This is why two of my four pillars address the internal processes that make it easier to cope with pain. We will get more into those pillars when we discuss the full framework in Chapter 7, but to give you a taste, recall the concept of the observer previously mentioned in Chapter 4. By allowing ourselves space to observe and respond, we can then employ the strategies discussed in Chapter 7 to cope with the experience of pain.

You do not - and should not - stop moving. Please keep moving in the best ways you can. Where other sources may provide you different advice, I promise that you will find a vibrant life on the other end of the skills I teach within my framework. After all, you have my lived experience and the lived experience of those I've worked with to bolster you through the learning process.

Inflammation

For better or worse, inflammation is the hallmark of chronic disease conditions.

What many don't understand is that there is both good and bad inflammation.

Good inflammation kicks in when we have a cut or a virus. Our body releases chemicals, nutrients, and hormones to the site of infection or injury and protects it via an inflammatory process. We've seen the swelling, the fluid, and the heat that comes with this acute inflammation. Without this process, our race would have died millions of years ago. Without the inflammatory process, we would die from even minor infections and injuries.

What happens is this acute inflammation can become chronic. That is a main contributing factor to chronic illness.

The regular inflammatory process produces chemicals, nutrients, and hormones, but this time it happens 24/7 - usually targeting a specific site - because your body thinks there is an injury or something off when, in reality, the cells are healthy.

This is what happens with diseases like multiple sclerosis. The inflammatory process attacks the myelin sheath of the nerve pathways. Rheumatoid arthritis is the inflammatory process attacking the linings of the joint capsules.

Chronic inflammation is on the rise for a few reasons, such as environmental hazards, but the biggest reason chronic inflammation is becoming more and more of a problem is our blood sugar levels.

Sugar is a poison to your system, and exercise is the natural antidote.

When you exercise, you use up the glucose in the bloodstream, and that is so helpful. When you exercise consistently over a long period of time, you rebalance the heightened sugar in the bloodstream (as long as you don't keep feeding yourself high sugar foods!)

Your muscles are metabolically active all hours of the day. Even while you are asleep, they are working, processing.

This is one reason sarcopenia comes to bite us when

we're older. The lessened muscle mass causes a reduction in the processing of glucose in the bloodstream, ultimately triggering the inflammatory response because of the high sugar content in your bloodstream. This is one reason strength training is so important as it builds up the size of our muscles.

Your body activates its natural process of dealing with a perceived threat and instead ends up attacking healthy cells in the body. This threat could be sugar, as discussed above, or heightened levels of cortisol and adrenaline from chronic stress.

No wonder inflammation is so prevalent in older people! Our natural aging process lends itself to multiple pathways all leading to chronic inflammation.

It's fascinating, and if you understand it, it becomes easier to work with and manage. The principles that build up the four pillars of my approach address these root causes of inflammation. Later in this book, I'll share practices you can use to lower your cortisol levels and, thus, lessen chronic inflammation.

Other Chronic Illnesses

Four out of five people over 65 have a chronic illness. That number is staggering!

What's more, *the majority of the people in this category have two or more chronic illnesses.*

It's awful to think of all of those people suffering. There are genetic factors and aging factors, but it's mostly due to lack of information and lifestyle choices.

For instance, a lot of women believe that heart disease is something that usually happens to men, *but it is the number one killer of women worldwide.* The problem is that the potential symptoms of a heart attack look very different in men and women.

We can get the traditional arm and chest pain but for many women, the more typical heart attack symptoms can come as a sense of unease and stomach cramps. There is a more visceral abdominal pain and a vague sense of nausea.

Type 2 diabetes is a huge problem among our population and can be managed with informed decisions about dieting, exercise, and lifestyle.

Dementia, including Alzheimer's Disease, is on the rise and is changing the lives of so many people. Hypertension (high blood pressure) is another that comes to mind from the clients in my classes. The list can sometimes feel like a living horror movie where you spin the wheel and wait for a doomed fate...

The importance of a holistic approach to wellness cannot be overstated here.

Management of a chronic illness or condition is possible! You can have more control in a situation you didn't get to choose.

Physical exercise is important, but is not the whole story. There are four pillars to my approach because these different aspects of wellness give you different techniques and tools that change your capacity to live your life in a much different way.

The combination of these pillars helps with inflammation so you can manage and/or improve the process of chronic illness. It addresses the strength and power of your muscles, the health of your cardiac system and your lung health, your cognitive functions, your thinking speed, your attention, and your memory. It also helps you overall in coping with and managing your experience of chronic illness.

More often than not, taking this proactive approach can lessen the impact - or in some cases get rid - of a chronic illness. Things like arthritis are degenerative and unable to be reversed, *but you can significantly lower the impact of arthritis on your life and slow its progression.* Experiences like obesity, type 2 diabetes, osteoporosis, some cancers, hypertension, and even heart disease, if caught and treated, can be ameliorated.

It's all about changing the relationship you have with chronic illness. Being open and inviting change will honestly impact your results more than the "woe is me" attitude. It comes down to resilience in three areas: your mind, body, and heart.

While we've discussed what happens in the body due to arthritis, inflammation, and chronic illness, it is important to remember the synchronicity and connection your mind, body, and heart have with each other.

Before we move on to the four pillars that allow you to age on your own terms (which you'll find in Chapter 7), I need to make one thing clear...

PART 2

The No Nonsense Approach to Controlling How You Age

Chapter 6

The #1 Ingredient You Need to Control How You Age

It's perfectly clear that the number one myth out there about getting older is wrong.

That myth is this: it is too late to make the changes you want.

So many of the women I work with don't understand the importance of being aerobically fit and strong as they age. Society feeds a belief that as you get older, you become less active and you become too old to try new things and should accept the slow down and let yourself go...

Absolutely not.

You need to understand that this is the best time to start getting fit and strong and mentally switched on, vibrant in body and brain.

What I teach here is *key to thriving and survival*. Our lives depend on our physical, cognitive, and emotional health.

It is not too late for you, and I am sad every time I hear that phrase uttered because I know that it's not true. If you feel like you're out of time, I would love to be able to guide and shift that belief. We all have the capacity to change our fitness and to change our strength, and we have to work out how that is best for you because we're all different.

This isn't about setting back the clock and marking time waiting for the final bell. It's about finding what works best for you and starting somewhere no matter how old you are.

The core of starting this journey is rooted in self-belief.

(Oh no, did she just say self-belief?)

Now, the general response to soft, squishy subjects like "self-belief" or "mindfulness" or even "self-compassion" is to roll your eyes and utter that loud 'T' sound of disapproval.

(Oh no, did she say mindfulness again?!)

That reaction makes sense. I get it. We grew up when "gurus" were bringing practices like meditation over from the East.

Stay with me for a minute. Let me demonstrate the difference between what we grew up with and what actually works in terms of these seemingly softer practices.

We witnessed the rise of meditation being brought from the East to the West in the sixties and seventies, particularly in America and Europe. There were some very influential names in this space that did so much good. They visited Buddhist monasteries in the East and learned about meditation, bringing back these practices to the mainstream of Western culture and society.

However, the essence of how these practices were taught to begin - the traditional approaches - clashed with our Western culture.

The instruction received was "clear your mind of thoughts," "have a mind that is a vacuum," "focus on your breath and empty your mind."

Now, this is actually impossible for us to accomplish given our society and culture. We have these minds that are thinking machines! Someone coming in and telling us to stop thinking, clear our minds of thoughts, and be at peace and relax is quite difficult.

The very real response was, "Oh God, I can't do that! I'm no good at that."

Most of us in the baby boomer generation had a negative reaction and initial experience with meditation. We are a straightforward generation. We just get in there and try and fix what is broken and don't complain about it - well, not out loud anyways. There's no time for all that emotional stuff, contemplation, and self-reflection. This just makes you weak and vulnerable.

We couldn't find the value in meditation because we were instructed in a way that was counterintuitive to our way of being.

Thankfully, there are people who have changed the language and understanding around the practice of meditation.

They have morphed the instruction around meditation and turned it into mindfulness (consequently, one of my four pillars).

Instead of trying to clear your mind, to stop thinking, the practice of mindfulness is more about being aware of your 'thinking machine.' Your mind.

So, we're not actually doing anything with our thoughts aside from stepping back and observing them. Each time we get distracted by our thinking machine (which is normal and will happen a lot in your practice!), you gently redirect your attention back to whatever it was that you are mindfully focusing on. Do this over and over again with each distraction that comes.

This distinction is not only much easier for us to accomplish but it also has more benefits than running around trying to stop the incessant stream of thoughts.

The incredible part is that this practice of self-belief actually affects you at a cellular level.

When you're self-critical, there is a degree of anxiety and stress happening in your body. You release adrenaline and cortisol in response to these thoughts and feelings. By this point in our history, there is a heap of evidence that cortisol hanging around in your body long-term is not good. It causes inflammation that can create diseases like Alzheimer's, heart disease, issues with blood vessels, some cancers, and high blood pressure.

Long-term cortisol and inflammation in the body is a major cause of chronic illness.

Believing in yourself and showing yourself compassion reduces these hormones and chronic inflammation which can reduce the likelihood of experiencing these significant health challenges. **In simple terms of longevity, self-belief is crucial.**

A singular act of self-kindness affects your very cells and how they function by virtue of this reduction in stress hormones. If you can bring this practice into your life as a habit of how you relate to yourself, then *you are doing one of the best things possible to keep the cellular integrity of your body intact.*

You can do this.

You can read all you want about exercise programs and diets, get all of the world's secrets about aging gracefully, and still fall short if you don't believe in your own ability to make changes.

There's a common belief that the problem with maintaining an exercise program is that people are lazy, don't have willpower, or are unmotivated.

Rubbish.

It's about the self-belief that you are worth the effort (and the fact that you may not be enjoying the exercise you're doing or getting the benefits you need or want from the exercise).

The truth is, you are not too old. You are not out of time. It's not too late.

You are capable. That is a fact. The four pillars of my method are based on principles that you can apply no matter your situation. In a sense, these pillars all work together to address the obstacles - self-imposed and external - you experience in your day-to-day life.

I know you may be dealing with a chronic illness like we just talked about in the last chapter. I know you have 50+ years of hearing how "that's just what happens when you get older."

I know I'm fighting an uphill battle here to get you on board with these softer concepts, but I am not going to stop. The book keeps going. I hope you can keep reading and digesting so you can make the best decision for yourself.

The four pillars of my method are based on years of research and work combining clinical psychology and fitness training. They are simple, and like many simple things, powerful.

Even if all you can do is read with reservations, I invite you to continue and encourage you to believe in the truth: it is not too late, and you can do this.

Understand that your mind (brain), body, and heart are interconnected (Chapter 4) and **believe in yourself and your ability to change**.

These two principles lay the foundation for the promise you came for: the no-nonsense approach to controlling how you age.

Chapter 7

The Four Pillar Method

Finally, the four pillars that allow you to age on your own terms and control the outcome of your aging experience.

Each of these pillars positively, productively, and constructively build off of each other. There's a synchronicity to how they work together. When you use the principles behind each pillar in your daily life, you become more grounded, healthy, and able to live life on your own terms.

The First Pillar: Exercise

My lived experience built this first pillar.

As a clinical psychologist, it could have been easy to intellectually understand the importance of physical health without hands-on expertise, but as you know from Chapter 2, that wasn't my journey!

Flourishing through my own health journey and becoming a fitness trainer were crucial to the longevity and capability I now experience as a 65-year-old woman.

Both Clinical Psychology and Professional Fitness Training have been an integral part of my life for 30+ years. As we learned in Chapter 4, the mind, body, and heart are forever connected.

My inquiring mind has turned physical exercise and education into an obsession. I am always learning the latest information and research about exercise and what I know is this: you can't just exercise. **You have to exercise effectively and sufficiently to truly impact your health.**

This doesn't mean the expectation is a rigorous workout or strict regimen. We need to find our own way of exercising. One that slots easily into our lives, one that we love, and one that gets the results we want and need.

Most people are active in some way, and you can keep doing what you are doing. Easy as that.

If you currently enjoy walking, that's great! I would encourage you to keep walking and slowly evolve your walking so it becomes what we would define as exercise. You don't have to call it exercise - you can still call it walking. Over time, it gradually morphs into the type of walking that will sustain your physical health.

Scientists and doctors are saying it is absolutely imperative that you exercise in a way that is effective, sufficient, and appropriate and that you do the right kind of exercise for your health.

This would be a good place to stop and define what "sustaining your physical health" looks like...

Except, that's actually up to you.

For example, I work with many women who suffer from arthritis.

As a refresher, arthritis happens in our joints, a joining of two bones or more, where there's a nice cushioning pad of cartilage, and muscles, ligaments, and tendons along with something called **synovial fluid**. This is a lubricating fluid that protects the joint by reducing friction when you move your joints. It also provides nutrients for the optimal function of the joint. Through the use of our joints over a long period of time, cartilage starts to wear down and we experience a reduction in synovial fluid.

Arthritis is essentially inflammation, pain, soreness, and stiffness in and around the joint and the various components that make up the joint.

I see arthritis go undiagnosed simply because we are afraid to go to the doctor. Good old juicy denial is much easier in the short-term, isn't it? But, there are things you can do to improve arthritis, and the sooner you know that's what's happening, the better.

The first thing your doctor will ask you is if you are exercising. Normally, the response is, "Of course not. It's too painful."

Here in Australia, the regular practice at this point is to refer the patient to an exercise physiologist, some-one who is trained to deal with and apply exercise to a chronic condition like arthritis or encourage them to find a personal fitness trainer or participate in an appropriate group class. In fact, many fitness trainers, myself included, can provide an individual program or group exercise class that will help manage arthritis.

Does it surprise you that exercise, something that can be uncomfortable or even painful, is the answer here?

The simple reason exercise is important is that if you don't move your body, the arthritis will get much worse.

If you stay still, the muscles around the joint become less powerful, strong, and supportive of your joint. If you buy into the negative arthritic mindset of, "I can't do that because I've got arthritis," then those muscles start to waste. Our muscles are already wasting due to something called sarcopenia. This is the reduction of muscle size and power as we age.

It's not just about muscle size and strength. It's about endurance and the ability of the muscle to do what it's designed to do. If you're not exercising - or even just moving - then it's going to fall away and the arthritis will get much worse because you lose the infrastructure around the joint in question.

Exercise, while challenging at times, actually protects the joint experiencing arthritis.

If you needed more of a reason to be open and embrace movement with arthritis, recall the reduction of synovial fluid in our initial description of what happens with arthritis.

When you exercise, you warm up the tissues in your joints, actually increasing the movement of your synovial fluid! When your joints become stiff, it's because that fluid becomes kind of sticky and doesn't flow around the joint as well as it could. Exercising essentially lubricates your joints and liquifies the stiff fluid, allowing it to cushion your joints more than it previously did.

It makes sense if you have stopped exercising and

moving due to arthritis. Arthritic joint pain hurts. Of course, the natural inclination is to stop doing something that hurts you. In fact, it seems like common sense that moving something that hurts could cause further injury.

What isn't understood is that the best way to help arthritis seems counterintuitive. If you are experiencing osteoarthritis and have the right guidance, the right support, and the right exercises and warmups, it's not necessarily going to hurt. It's alright to feel a bit of discomfort. That's something we have to learn to cope with (continue with the pillars below).

For someone with arthritis, "sustaining physical health" can simply mean continuing to move and work the affected joints. For others, "sustaining physical health" might mean something different.

Health can be very esoteric.

You know that your heart will be stronger and your joints won't ache as bad, but what does being healthy actually mean to you? What would being more healthy look like in your life? What activities would you be able to continue to do?

The principle at play here is less a step-by-step system and more a philosophy that aligns your actions and choices to the life you want in your older years.

Make it less about the health benefits - because those

will absolutely follow physical exercise - and make it about how your life will be different in the future. Why is it important to have a good heart, less creaky joints, or the ability to walk at a brisk pace for more than 5 minutes?

For some, it's wanting to take advantage of the beautiful scenery while traveling. Others simply want to keep up with their grandkids! Others still want to be able to carry their groceries from the car and into the kitchen. Socializing and a passionate hobby like cooking, gardening, dog walking, writing, and the like all require a healthy and functioning body to enjoy.

When you workout or gradually up your walking pace, focus on this 'why.' What are these health benefits going to mean in terms of how you are going to live and age through the rest of your years on this planet?

Quick-start Exercise Ideas

- Go on a walk around your neighborhood (bonus points for inviting a friend to walk with you).

- While cooking, practice balancing on one leg or doing a few squats.

The Second Pillar: Cognition

About fifteen years ago, I lost a very beloved auntie to Alzheimer's Disease.

She was the life and soul of the party, and she would have been 95 this year. She was the most amazing, vibrant, beautiful woman.

Yet, Alzheimer's doesn't discriminate. She succumbed to the disease, and both of her daughters now experience Alzheimer's as well.

Now, I'm not saying you're going to get Alzheimer's. Perhaps you have had a similar experience of a family member or loved one decline in this way. My closest cousin, one of my auntie's daughters mentioned before, lives across Australia from me. I call her every month and I see the deterioration in her condition.

I am reminded of how vital it is that if you've got the know-how, the lived personal experience, the information, the skills, the personality, and the aptitude to create a difference in people's lives around cognitive health - you've just got to do it.

This is the biggest reason I encourage anyone and everyone to take care of their cognitive health (their brains): to help families reduce the possibility of getting Alzheimer's. If it's not possible to stop it altogether, then we ameliorate the symptoms and significantly slow the speed of decline.

I have the lived experience of seeing firsthand how devastating that can be for the person experiencing the disease and for the family members involved. I will never cease to teach those in my classes and circles of influence the education and actions needed to maintain your cognitive health.

While physical exercise has been shown to improve brain health, recent research strongly suggests that you have to introduce specific cognitive activities while exercising to fully benefit.

Targeted cognitive exercises whilst moving, whilst exercising, are another crucial pillar layered in my health approach for women as they age.

As we get older, our cognitions, the activity of our brains, becomes compromised through the natural aging process. This does not mean we are all at the mercy of getting Dementia, including Alzheimer's Disease, *but we do need to keep our brains active to age on our own terms.*

During my initial Brain Health Training certification, Dr. Ryan Glatt presented significant research on the needed benefits of combining exercise and cognitive training. Through each recertification of this training, the evidence and importance of intentionally exercising your brain while exercising your body became more clear. This training was further reinforced by my recent certification as an Alzheimer's Disease Fitness Specialist.

There is a desperate need to keep working our brains. You'll have seen the push in brain training apps and online games specifically designed to support the maintenance of cognitive resources.

You'll see how I combine specific cognitive exercises with physical activity in the videos I shared with you upon your purchase of this book. (These videos came as a 'Thank You' em   .

As you try these exercises out (please do!), you'll feel a greater sense of self-efficacy, of control, of mastery, and of resilience that you are doing all you can based on the latest research to help how your brain ages. The actual science of delaying cognitive decline - or stopping it altogether - is where the cognitive aspect of my program comes from.

Even if you don't join my full program, keep doing the cognitive things you are drawn to, like crosswords, Sudoku puzzles, or learning a language or a musical instrument - but also social connection and maintaining a sense of purpose. All of these things done daily, even if in small doses, can go an incredible way toward maintaining your cognitive health as you age.

Quick-start Cognition Ideas

- Spell your spouse's or friend's name backwards with your nose in the air while walking around the house.

- Tap your head (with both hands), then clap your hands, then pat your tummy twice (with both hands). Speed this up and then reverse the sequence.

The Third Pillar: Mindfulness

We touched on this concept back in Chapter 4. Mindfulness is the ability to stand back and be the observer of your thoughts, feelings, and experiences.

Where mindfulness can trigger thoughts of meditation - and your uneasiness around meditation - recall the difference between what we saw in the sixties and what we experience now as discussed back in Chapter 6.

Mindfulness is gently redirecting your attention back to a central point of focus.

You can do this while walking. You can do this sitting in your favorite chair while stroking your cat (or dog).

You can do this while sitting outside watching the clouds roll by.

You can even do this in the middle of a hectic work day or family celebration. ***Mindfulness enhances your experience of the present moment.***

Mindfulness is what allows you to feel an emotion and not be overcome by it or your reaction to it. It's what allows you to accept pain - physical or otherwise - and not shrink or become bitter from it.

The pillar of mindfulness is what allows you to age with grace and gratitude.

Back in Chapter 4, we discussed the concept of becoming the observer of your own experiences.

If that analogy doesn't resonate with you, try looking at yourself as if you are your very own friend.

If you find yourself in a dispute with your colleague, neighbor, or a family member, pause, step back, and reflect. How would you advise a friend to react in your shoes? What would you teach to your children around the table at dinner?

This shift in perspective is essentially what you do when you become the observer.

You are no longer ruled by the moment, no longer hijacked by old patterns. Instead, you gain the ability to apply the wisdom of your many lived experiences to each day and each event. This ability allows you to live with appreciation, clarity, and depth.

When you live with mindfulness, you are more aware of what your body tells you, more aware of what your heart expresses, and more aware of your thoughts. With more self-awareness, you cultivate the capacity to monitor and manage your life, especially your life now when things can change very quickly.

Mindfulness is the gentle pillar that boosts the effectiveness of exercise, contributes to cognitive toughness, and cradles self-compassion.

Quick-start Mindfulness Ideas

- Go for a walk and notice the colors and shapes of all the objects you pass.

- When you recognize you're lost in thought, say, "They are just thoughts." Bring your attention back to what you were doing, noticing what you can hear around you.

The Fourth Pillar: Self-Compassion

The same is true with self-compassion as it is with mindfulness.

Many women in our age range believe that self-compassion is a load of garbage; a self-help, psycho-babble, hippy thing from the sixties and seventies that will make you selfish and weak.

I would not be surprised if you saw my fourth pillar and thought, "Oh God, she's talking about self-compassion. I'm out."

There's something about showing ourselves kindness and self-love that's uncomfortable. Addressing emotional health is often taboo among our generation.

I'm here to share with you the hard truth: your emotional well-being is an essential part to your aging process.

We deal with so much in these years. There is a constant busyness being sandwiched between caretaking for our parents, our children, and our grandchildren. There is pain in loss as we say goodbye to good friends and parents who pass on. There is physical pain from our aging bodies and frustration at the changes in our communities and governments.

The list goes on.

Any one of those things can cause significant emotional distress.

But, there's another side to our emotions that doesn't get our attention nearly as often.

How do you feel when you forget to buy something at the supermarket? How do you feel when your grandson tells you about his new Pokémon game and you realize you can't understand a word he's saying? How do you feel when you can't open a jar of honey when you could last week?

What do you say to yourself when you fall short while hosting a gathering because your energy is depleted?

Most of us give ourselves a hard time. We tell ourselves that it's time to just get on with it and deal with it. That was how we were raised, after all.

This is nothing compared to what our mothers experienced. They were always able to keep a hot, three-course meal on the table for dinner after working during the day and maintaining a clean home. They always came last and never complained about it. If they did, no one listened anyway.

Even though we have the benefit of self-help books and life coaches who have taught us to be nice to ourselves, *we still see ourselves as falling short.*

This emotional standpoint can undercut every other gain you experience from the other three pillars.

Self-compassion isn't about being soft and squishy with no accountability or direction; it's about giving yourself a break. *This pillar is crucial to your all-around health and well-being.*

The women I talk with through my program confide that they feel guilty when they want to do something for themselves. They say it feels bad, uncomfortable, or downright selfish to put themselves first. Everyone else's needs are more important. When others are sorted, then there's time for themselves... but by then, you're so exhausted you can't do anything.

As a woman of 65, a psychologist, a fitness trainer, and a mindfulness trainer – I am here to tell you that self-compassion is not an option as you get older. It is a matter of survival.

The good news is this: developing self-compassion is not learning how to be selfish or self-indulgent. Self-compassion is about becoming self-aware and assertive.

Just like mindfulness, it's a skill. All it takes is a bit of practice.

Thankfully, there's significant research on how you can bring self-compassion into your life while still maintaining your important relationships and lists of tasks you want to do. Self-compassion brings the much needed balance you might feel is missing from your life.

Practicing this skill can be as simple as recognizing that you're struggling with your day without being harsh with yourself. It can be as simple as seeing that you're busy and saying to yourself, "What I'm doing here is important. I need to spend this time looking after my [mother/father/grandkids], but I've got this. I'm going to sit here with them and enjoy this time with them."

The essence of this pillar involves mindfulness, self-kindness, and common humanity.

It doesn't have to be going for a massage or a hot bath. This essence is best demonstrated in a moment of frustration. Instead of avoiding the feeling, shoving it down, or blowing up, you can say, "I've got some frustration here in my body. I'm going to be mindful of that. It's an experience I'm having. This isn't who I am. I'm going to offer myself some kindness and give myself a break. This is just what I need to do right now. It's not about me being wrong. I don't have to take this frustration personally. This is just part of being a human being on planet earth."

This is called the self-compassion break. You're not failing yourself if you acknowledge struggle. You are not falling short when responding with gentleness to an internal hardship.

You are affecting your very cellular structure (Chapter 6) and allowing yourself good mental and physical health.

It just makes you feel better! Negative emotional and mental health experiences are ameliorated with consistent self-compassion because it does wonders to quieten our internal critics and reorient our focus to something more pleasant.

As we learned in Chapter 4, our minds, bodies, and hearts are inseparably connected. Self-compassion directly affects each aspect of our being.

Quick-start Self Compassion Ideas

- When you notice you have made a mistake, pause for a moment and ask yourself why that mistake made sense. Were you distracted or talking on the phone? Are you feeling incredibly tired today? The "it makes sense" approach allows you grace without excusing the mistake or beating yourself up.

- When you're struggling with something, place a hand on your heart, your tummy,

or your cheek. This soothes the anguish
of the experience.

Exercise. Cognitive Training. Mindfulness. Self-compassion.

These are the tenants of connecting your mind, body, and heart.

These are the practices that will allow you to take control of how you age.

I will help you through the first steps of practicing these principles in Part 3. But first, there are some critical components that are important to have in place...

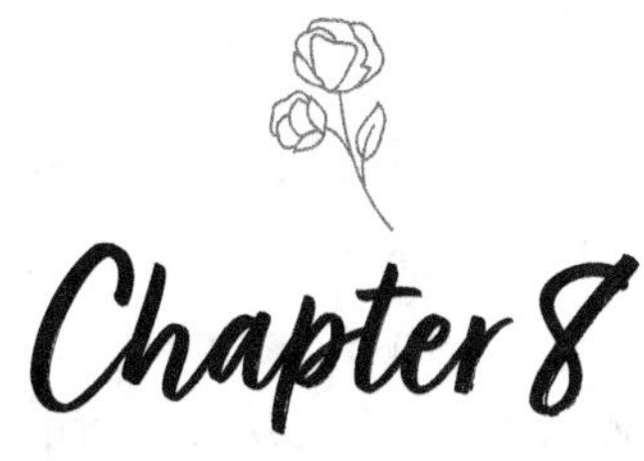

Chapter 8

Critical Components to Aging Well

Applying the four pillars of exercise, cognitive training, mindfulness, and self-compassion will radically change the way you age, ushering in a vibrant way of life.

Below are a few supports to elevate your experiences in these four areas.

Diet

To be totally and 100% clear, there is no diet restriction to making this method work for you.

I encourage you to be mindful of what you eat. I call this *intuitive eating*. My approach is rooted in self-compassion, that open and understanding relationship you have with yourself, where you naturally eat well because you respect and honor your body and brain. When you relate to yourself in this way, you start to gravitate towards eating styles or habits that are akin to looking after yourself.

Your diet is incredibly important because it determines what fuel you give to your body. As we know, body, mind, and heart are all connected. Feeding your body good food will positively influence not only your physicality but your brain power, your mental energy, and your emotional stability.

I'm not going to dictate what you need to eat and avoid, have you schedule your meals, or count your macros. Those are generally stipulations in a weight loss program, and this is not about weight loss. It's about self-efficacy and empowerment while you age. Healthy eating is my aim for you. You can eat in a way that resonates with you and enjoy the benefits of eating well.

If you're not sure where to start, I suggest you find a program that a friend has tried and loved, preferably a method that is designed and validated by someone like a medical practitioner with a track record of success in their field. The other option is to get a referral from your General Practitioner to a registered dietitian or nutritionist. They are trained to take into account your lifestyle and any health related data when helping you figure out the best diet for you.

Among my favorites is the Mediterranean diet. It's highly recommended by many medical professionals as one of the best diets for brain and body health.

This is the diet in several "Blue Zones" around the globe. These zones have been studied ad nauseum because they have the highest number of healthy centenarians (people over a hundred years old!) From these studies alone, the Mediterranean diet always comes up as a diet for longevity, cognitive health, and physical health.

However you approach your diet, I encourage you to be mindful of what you eat and how you eat. Ask yourself if you're giving your body the nutrition it needs, if you're sacrificing a healthy colon for your favorite sweet, if you could counteract painful reflux by eating smaller portions, etc.

Every *body* is different. Intuitive eating, mindful eating, is about being aware of your own body, how it reacts to the food you're eating, and what differences in an approach might be helpful for your specific situation.

Social Connection

Loneliness is a huge problem with our generation,

particularly in this age ruled by the internet where people are becoming more socially isolated.

This is an area we need to make a purposeful effort in to continue with our friendships. Social connection is important to our mental and emotional health and it requires effort and energy to maintain.

As with a diet, this can be done however it best resonates with you. Track down a group exercise class. Volunteer in your community. Join a book club. Spend quality time with your kids and grandkids. However this best fits into your life and fills you up, make the effort.

In my program, I am very big on having streamed group sessions so my clients have that sense of community. We have a "coffee hour" after some of our exercise sessions to chat and connect with each other.

It takes energy to make friends. It takes effort to maintain those close connections. This reminds you of your 'why' to remain fit and healthy. It's hard to make choices about healthy things to eat, whom you're going to engage with, or how you're going to show up in your life when it's all you can do to simply get out of bed in the morning.

Recall back to the beginning of this book where we discussed the importance of finding your 'why' to keeping fit and healthy. Your motivation, or 'why,' also applies to social connection as it is one aspect of being whole and healthy.

Social connection is easiest to keep up with, and does the most good, when it's *meaningful*. That can look different for everyone. What makes for meaningful connection in your life? Try to identify a few bullet points that define what this concept means for you.

The four pillars combined with the understanding of a connected mind, body, and heart is the springboard to taking control of how you age.

Momentum

If there's one thing I hope you do after reading this book, it's to **keep doing what you're doing**.

Don't stop using the brain training app your niece told you to download. Stimulate your brain in whatever way you've been enjoying.

Don't replace your current walking routine. Keep doing what fits into your life and then expand from there.

If a 'Words With Friends' competition with your son keeps your mind nimble and sharp, there's no need to stop and try one of the other things mentioned in this book. Even if you join one of my programs, it's all about continuing to do what works for you.

If you're not engaging in the four pillars, then think about ways to introduce them into your life. The next section of this book will outline ways to get started in these areas. Feel free to use these exercises if you need to add them, or leave them behind if they don't work for you. ***The important thing is to incorporate the principles of exercise, cognition, mindfulness, and self-compassion into your daily life***.

Once you start, your brain starts to wake up and get energized. It's like a big sponge. The more you tickle it, the more it picks up and the more it wants! Whilst my program is brilliant and the thirty minutes three times a week is wonderful, why not make the most out of your brain being fired up and hungry for activity?

What novel and fun things do you enjoy? If that's difficult to answer, look back to your childhood. What have you done in your life that made you feel alive? Was there anything you weren't allowed to do as a kid that you thought might be interesting or exciting?

Take what works for you and leave the rest behind. Start somewhere and build from there. Engage with what resonates with you, and the momentum you build will be more powerful than any one-size-fits-all approach.

PART 3

Start Today

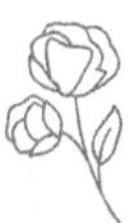

Beginnings of Exercise

For first steps in exercise, there are two starting points I recommend based on what works best for your current situation.

1. If you already engage in a physical activity, like walking, then keep doing that. Start challenging yourself while you're on your walk to take it up a notch for 10, 20, or 30 seconds. See if you can walk a little faster up a steep hill, introduce some shuffles in your step, or jogs momentarily if your body is comfortable with that. Extend yourself gradually as you continue to engage in your chosen activity. Gauge how your body responds in terms of health and fitness just by stepping a little bit out of your comfort zone. Use that information to determine how you can push yourself a little bit each time you are active.

2. If you are looking for a place to start with exercise, I invite you to check out the emails you got along with the purchase of this book or the videos within your membership area. I share exercises that are designed for women like you and me! I include the four pillars in each workout. It's a great way to get started if you don't currently have a physical activity you like to engage in and a wonderful way to continue being active even if you already have a preferred exercise.

Remember, the important aspect here is to keep the momentum of being active. Why do you want a healthy body? Is it so you can get on the floor with your grandkids? Is it so you can finally take that European walking trip you've always wanted to? Focus on your 'why' when you engage in your chosen physical activity to ground yourself and remain motivated to continue with consistency and compassion.

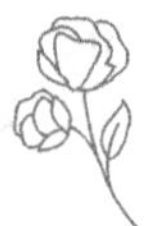

Beginnings of Cognitive Training

There are a few different streams you can use to stimulate your brain.

The first that generally comes to mind is some sort of online brain training program. I personally like to use CogniFit, but there are others like BrainHQ. These services are advertised as brain training, designed to help keep our minds nimble. They can work really well!

The one complaint some researchers have with brain training games is something called the rehearsal bias. Your brain is incredible at finding patterns and forming pathways, and some of these online training apps lend themselves to familiarization. The brain gets good at recognising the pattern and it's not necessarily improving cognitive capacities. If you use one of these online platforms, keep going with them as they're great - but it's important to keep the brain involved in additional new and novel tasks as well.

The second stream I highly recommend is specifically learning a new language or a musical instrument. These two activities come up in research again and again as being very effective to maintaining cognitive abilities. Often, older people have some sort of regret tied to one or both of these. Perhaps you played piano as a child and stopped playing when life got busy. Maybe you learned a bit of German in high school and always thought it would be cool to learn more.

You don't have to go out of your way to learn a language or instrument if that doesn't resonate with you. For example, learning a new language is not something in my repertoire. If you decide to learn a language or musical instrument, the inherent challenge will fire up your brain in new and novel ways with each new song or phrase you learn.

There are many different ways to stimulate your brain.

For instance, there are things like word games, crossword puzzles, memory games, reading books, etc. These are very cognitive specific, meaning they only target one or two cognitive abilities (or what's called cognitive domains) like memory or mental focus. Something like a musical instrument, foreign language, or the cognitive training included in my program target a range of different cognitive functions.

Whether cognitive specific or more general, none of it is wasted! It's a good activity to do and certainly better than not doing anything. When you're fully engaged in a jigsaw puzzle, there is still a benefit when your attention is focused and you're using your brain to decide how you're going to do a particular activity.

Of course, if you decide to join my program or follow me on social media, you will find the dual tasking of cognition and exercise in each class I lead. This is an excellent way to sharpen and maintain cognitive function.

Like the exercise section, I would recommend extending yourself a bit. Keep doing what you're doing and look for ways you can incorporate new brain training processes and novel activities into your life.

Beginnings of Mindfulness

Mindfulness is about how you relate to what's happening and, in particular, your thoughts. It's not about clearing your mind and not thinking of anything. It's about being aware of your thoughts.

It's much easier to experience than explain.

A surprising way to practice mindfulness is to recognise when you're getting distracted. Distraction is a wonderful opportunity to practice mindfulness!

Next time you're cooking dinner, focus on the food, your actions, and the recipe. Note when your mind wanders. Without judgment, take note of what you're thinking about. Was there an appointment with your doctor that left some lingering questions? Are you excited for a family gathering happening this weekend?

Gently redirect your thoughts back to cooking.

You can do this while breathing, crocheting, walking, etc. Any activity can lend itself to mindfulness because you need only be present and aware of your thoughts and gently redirect your attention back to your chosen activity.

Another way of practicing mindfulness can happen when you're still. (And no - you don't have to sit cross-legged on the floor!) You can sit in a chair, lay in your bed, or do whatever is comfortable to you. Now, focus on the physical sensations present. What are the contact points of your body on the chair? What does your breath feel like entering your body and leaving it?

This is also a practice in mindfulness. You can feel where your back touches the chair. You can feel your head bobbing around. The physical awareness of your own body is a wonderful grounding technique, especially when you feel your thoughts are getting away from you.

Beginnings of Self-Compassion

We touched on this earlier, but I need you to know that self-compassion is okay. In fact, it's crucial to your health and well-being.

Having self-compassion as a foundation offers you the energy to be more available for other people in your life. Its reciprocal relationship improves everything it touches.

You don't need an in-depth understanding to get started.

A really good place to start is with a practice called 'the supportive touch' where you offer yourself a touch that is synonymous with care and warmth. An appropriate, supportive touch, like placing your hand over your heart, feels comfortable.

When I was a child, I would walk around and see a lot of the Italian and Greek immigrants that came here to Australia in the sixties. I was particularly touched by the lovely, warm, older women.

I noticed that they were usually dressed all in black and would often place a hand over their hearts. And, of course, I asked my mum why they were doing that. Now, she didn't explain it in terms of mindfulness or self-compassion like we are discussing here, but I remember her answer, "Well, I think her husband has died or she's lost another loved one and she's comforting herself. She wears black out of respect for those who have died."

This stuck with me through nursing school and my psychology degree. Mindfulness and self-compassion weren't taught then, but this memory always intrigued me.

Later in my life, at 60 years old, I remember my daughter saying to me, "Wow mom! You're officially an old woman."

"What do you mean?" I said.

"Well, you're touching your heart a lot. That's an old woman thing."

(She was joking with me, of course, as she knew about my memory of the women dressed in black. Those older women folk who needed comfort due to a loss in their life.)

Without recognising it, I had started placing my hand on my heart in a way to offer myself compassion. It's kind of like saying "you're hurting" or "this is difficult," and immediately my hand (or sometimes) go to my heart.

This practice is about embracing that you need warmth and nurturing, that you need that kindness and the reflection that you've been in pain or hurting because of something in your life, and that you need a supportive touch.

It's a great way to ground your stress response, especially when there's no one else around to give you a hug. Immediately, the cortisol, the adrenaline, falls away and you can be grounded in that sense of caring for yourself.

I know that out of all of the tasks I've given in this book, this might sound the strangest. I encourage you to give it a try. Place your hand over your heart and hold it there for a moment. Be there for yourself. Show yourself compassion and kindness.

Conclusion

If you bought this book, there's something within you that wants something different in your life.

There's something that niggles at you; that causes some discomfort or ill-at-ease-ness regarding the future and how it might look for you. This can start a cycle of more angst and worry that affects your body, your mind, and your heart.

If there's a disquiet there, an emptiness or an ache to have as much control and artistic license around what your future is going to look like... you have the foundation for your solution in your hands!

Tinged with these emotions is hopefully some excitement surrounding the possibility of creating a different relationship with yourself and that you can relate to your thoughts and emotions in a different way.

You can live your life with openness to the idea that *you can age on your own terms* instead of bowing to the negativity, the judgment, and the "shoulds," "cant's," and "musts."

Your life is your own. Your aging doesn't have to look like anyone else's.

If what you've read has settled within you, I invite you to go deeper. Explore. Go play! Decide what is going to work for you. Find what resonates with you.

If you'd like to work with me or see what I'm about, please reach out to me here: *http://bit.ly/4br7lBz*

Remember, it is the understanding that your mind, body, and heart are intertwined and self-belief that will pave the way for you to adopt exercise, cognitive training, mindfulness, and self-compassion into your life. These pillars, these tools, will allow you to live with grace and self-efficacy, fully staring aging in the face - and then having the skills to enjoy yourself and keep doing what you do.

With hope,

Penelope Lane

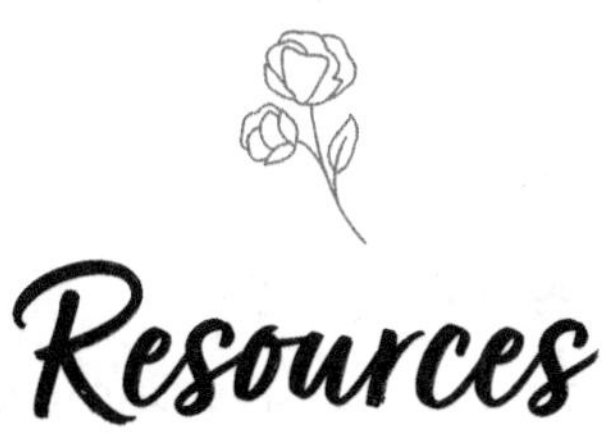

Resources

Locate all of your bonus material connected to this book in your Fit & Fabulous membership area.

You can find Kristen Neff's work here:
https://self-compassion.org/

Penelope's Favorite Mediterranean Recipes

- **Winter Evening Meal: Black Bean Brain-power Booster**
  (Suitable for 2 people)

  Ingredients:

  2 tbsp. olive oil

  2 sticks celery - finely chopped

1 medium carrot - finely chopped

1 medium beetroot shredded

1 small broccoli head

1 cup garden peas (fresh or frozen)

1 medium tomato

1 cup black beans

3 cups vegetable stock

3 cups cooked, mashed pumpkin or butternut squash

5 cups finely chopped kale

Ground black pepper to taste

Fresh garden herbs you love as a seasoning

Handful of pumpkin seeds

Method:

1. Pour olive oil in a large saucepan and cook chopped celery, carrots, and shredded beetroot for about 3 or so minutes.

2. Add broccoli, garden peas, and tomato, and cook a further 3 or so minutes.

3. Add stock and black beans. Heat till liquid starts to bubble.

4. Add kale, cooked pumpkin, and pepper. Cook till it resembles a kind of thick soup.

5. Add garden herbs and stir in for a few minutes.

6. Pour into plates with pumpkin seeds sprinkled on top.

If you want some good, wholesome grains with this, add cooked brown rice to your liking.

It can also be served with a wholesome wholegrain bread.

Oh... and a little bit of butter on that bread - why not, indeed!

- **Summer Evening Meal: Summer Salad Surprise**
(Suitable for 2 people)

Ingredients:

4 cups of any vegetable you like (chopped or shredded). You want a good selection with a range of different colours.

What I use:

Kale, carrots, beetroot, celery, spinach, red pepper, cabbage (green & purple), mushrooms and tomatoes.

1/2 cup or more of favourite olives

1/2 cup or more of feta cheese cubes

1 tbsp. olive oil

Juice of a small lime

3 tsp. balsamic vinegar

Salt and pepper to taste

1/2 tsp. honey (melted)

1/2 cup or more of any kind of chopped nuts: I use walnuts, cashews, and almonds.

Fresh garden herbs you love as a seasoning

Method:

1. Place all the chopped or shredded vegetables in your favourite salad bowl. Keep in fridge till you're ready to eat.

2. To make the salad dressing: combine the olive oil, lime juice, balsamic vinegar, salt, pepper, and honey and stir together.

3. When ready to serve, add the olives and feta cheese to the prepared vegetables. Pour the dressing over the other ingredients and mix them together.

4. Sprinkle the chopped nuts over the contents of the bowl and garnish with your favourite garden fresh herbs.

For protein, you can add your favourite legume. Sometimes I have it as is and other times I add 1/2 cup kidney beans per serving.

If you prefer meat, add your choice of cooked meat or fish.

It can also be served with a wholesome wholegrain bread.

Oh... and a little bit of butter on that bread - why not, indeed!

About the Author

Penelope Lane is an expert in fitness, psychology, cognitive health, and mindfulness.

As a Fitness Trainer, Clinical Psychologist, and Mindfulness Teacher, she has been helping women improve their fitness, strength, mobility, brainpower, and emotional health for more than 34 years.

She is a certified Personal Trainer and Clinical Psychologist with further qualifications in:

- Brain Health Training
- Group Exercise Training
- Alzheimer's Disease Fitness
- Older Adult Fitness
- Menopause Weight Loss Coaching
- Group Coaching

- Functional Training
- Mindfulness Teacher Training

From the fun of aerobics in the 80s to clinical psychology and nursing experience, to a passion for cognitive health and participating in CrossFit, she brings a vibrant mix of lively enthusiasm and serious, research-based training to activate the body and brain together.

For most of her youth, Penelope Lane was not a fit or healthy person. She struggled to find a health routine that made her feel vibrant and motivated. Everything changed when she became pregnant at 30 and realised she had to look after more than her own health. Through a mix of therapy, mindfulness, and family support, Penelope began a radical lifestyle change.

It was joining a boot camp in Perth, led by an ex-SAS soldier, that grew her love for group fitness. Reaching the elite squad, she realised how motivating and enjoyable group training could be.

Throughout her fitness journey, she has practised as a Clinical Psychologist and Nurse. On the side, she was a fitness instructor running group training and boot camps. Her unique approach to health is the culmination of her lifelong journey – from struggling with health and wellness to embracing physical and cognitive strength; a journey that saw her run her first half marathon at the age of 61!

Combining years of experience in psychology and fitness, she has designed a program to support women over 50 to unlock their best physical, cognitive, and emotional health. She is committed to helping others like herself to find their strength, vibrancy, confidence, and independence as older adults.

Get in touch with Penelope here:
http://bit.ly/4br7lBz

References

Ali, Nawab et al. "The Effects of Dual-Task Training on Cognitive and Physical Functions in Older Adults with Cognitive Impairment; A Systematic Review and Meta-Analysis." *The Journal of Prevention of Alzheimer's Disease* (2022): 1-12. https://www.semanticscholar.org/paper/The-Effects-of-Dual-Task-Training-on-Cognitive-and-Ali-Tian/ce1caf9ecf1f4a51d347c6dc-348d309a7cd0159c. Accessed May 2023.

Castaño Luz Albany Arcila, Castillo de Lima Vivian, et al. "Resistance Training Combined With Cognitive Training Increases Brain Derived Neurotrophic Factor and Improves Cognitive Function in Healthy Older Adults." *Frontiers in Psychology, Volume 13, 2022.* https://www.frontiersin.org/articles/10.3389/fpsyg.2022.870561. Accessed May 2023.

Gheysen, F., Poppe, L., DeSmet, A. et al. "Physical activity to improve cognition in older adults: can physical activity programs enriched with cognitive challenges enhance the effects? A systematic review and meta-analysis." *Int J Behav Nutr Phys Act 15, 63 (2018).* https://doi.org/10.1186/s12966-018-0697-x. Accessed April 2023.

Lauenroth, A., Ioannidis, A.E. & Teichmann, B. "Influence of combined physical and cognitive training on cognition: a systematic review." *BMC Geriatr 16, 141 (2016)*. https://doi.org/10.1186/s12877-016-0315-1. Accessed May 2023.

Torre, Marta Maria, and Jean-Jacques Temprado. "A review of combined training studies in older adults according to a new categorization of conventional interventions." *Frontiers in Aging Neuroscience 13 (2022): 808539*. https://www.frontiersin.org/articles/10.3389/fnagi.2021.808539. Accessed June 2023.

Qiang Zhou, Hongchang Yang, Quanfu Zhou, Hongyao Pan. "Effects of cognitive motor dual-task training on stroke patients: A RCT-based meta-analysis." *Journal of Clinical Neuroscience, Volume 92, 2021, Pages 175-182, ISSN 0967-5868*, https://doi.org/10.1016/j.jocn.2021.08.009. Accessed June 2023.

Varela-Vásquez LA, Minobes-Molina E, Jerez-Roig J. "Dual-task exercises in older adults: A structured review of current literature." *J Frailty Sarcopenia Falls. 2020 Jun 1;5(2):31-37*. doi: 10.22540/JFSF-05-031. PMID: 32510028; PMCID: PMC7272776. Accessed June 2023.

Zhu, Xinyi, et al. "The more the better? A meta-analysis on effects of combined cognitive and physical intervention on cognition in healthy older adults." *Ageing*

Research Reviews 31 (2016): 67-79. *https://www.sci-encedirect.com/science/article/pii/S1568163716301593*. Accessed May 2023.

Gheysen, F., Poppe, L., DeSmet, A. et al. "Physical activity to improve cognition in older adults: can physical activity programs enriched with cognitive challenges enhance the effects? A systematic review and meta-analysis." *Int J Behav Nutr Phys Act 15, 63 (2018).* *https://doi.org/10.1186/s12966-018-0697-x*

www.ingramcontent.com/pod-product-compliance
Lightning Source LLC
Chambersburg PA
CBHW070710250726
48662CB00001B/347